Pressing
RESET
for the
Parkinson's
Warriors

ᕼriginal strength

Original strength

Pressing RESET for the Parkinson's Warriors

Published by OS Press - Fuquay-Varina, NC

Contributor:
Ginny Scaduto, Certified Personal Trainer & Holistic Wellness Coach Specializing in Parkinson's Advocacy & Senior Fitness, Original Strength Certified Pro fitnessforwardmethod.com

Photagragaphy by: LaneBenson_photography

ISBN: 979-8-9865860-6-9 (Paperback)

Thank you to JETLAUNCH.net for editing and book design.

Introduction

"Movement is medicine for people with Parkinson's" is a fact that is continuously emphasized by most Parkinson's Medical Professionals, Support Groups and Research Organizations. While there is no cure YET, there is plenty of hope and progress being made in ways to slow progression and improve the day-to-day quality of life for people with Parkinson's. **And that journey can begin right here for you, by learning to Press RESET.**

Whether you are newly diagnosed or have been living with Parkinson's Disease for some time, this booklet was written to empower you with tools that can help you take more control over your health and well-being, and to help you to maintain your independence.

It is encouraging that the medical community, and all of the Parkinson's support organizations, acknowledge and promote the importance of movement to manage symptoms of the disease. The Michael J. Fox Foundation states it this way: Exercise is one of the most powerful treatments for Parkinson's Disease (PD). They go on to detail the positive impact of mitigating both motor and non-motor skill symptoms to include anxiety and sleep disorders.

At Original Strength we know that the body was designed to allow us to do **what** we need to do **when** we need to do it. This design includes a nervous system that has the ability to remember the developmental movement sequence that we were born with and that keeps us functional each day.

Our bodies were meant to be strong and capable throughout our lifetimes and while that may sound counter-intuitive if you are currently living with PD, the fact is that our bodies were designed to endure life and *all* of its challenges.

Recognizing that Parkinson's is a very complex and challenging condition, this information may help you to not only slow down progression, but to also help reduce pain and rigidity. It may help you to improve your balance. It may help you to become physically and mentally stronger overall. It may even help you to reduce anxiety and regain a curiosity and passion for living as you generate a few more smiles.

Yes, life happens. Accidents happen, injuries happen and diseases happen, but the body was made to heal and prevent injuries if it is moving and operating properly. This means we should not be limited by our current physical and mental condition - and with time, patience, positivity and consistency of effort - we don't have to be. If we can reclaim the way we were designed to move, we can restore strength, mobility, balance and power. Mobility that was once lost can return, pain can be alleviated and we can even restore our ability to focus, remember, interpret and analyze information the way that we used to; all through moving the way we were designed to move.

When we press RESET, our bodies respond at the speed of our nervous system. This can happen instantaneously for some, or it can take longer for others, but it will happen. That is why re-learning the way we were designed to move can help restore health and vitality.

Medical Disclaimer: It is important to note that we are not here to diagnose or treat any medical or physical disorder. This is meant to be a guide to restoring healthy functionality and should not supersede any medical advice from your doctor or other health professionals that you work with. Do not move into pain. Pain is an alarm system telling your body that something is or may be wrong and needs to be respected. Our bodies compensate and move very differently when we are in pain. As we move more, and better, your body should improve but if you cannot perform the movements in this guide without pain then seek a medical professional.

Pressing
RESET

We call this Original Strength

This is the strength we were created to have throughout our lifetime before PD movement disorders took over. This is the strength and mobility that allows us to live a better life, independently the way we want to. This is the strength that gives us the freedom to move and the ability to enjoy life. These qualities always live inside of us and can be released when we move according to our design.

In this booklet, we are going to demonstrate how to **press the reset button** on our body and move the way we were designed to so we can work towards restoring the Original Strength (OS) we were meant to have.

Our hope is that it will give you a fresh perspective and help you to remember **how good it feels to feel good.**

We Start from Good

No matter where you are right now, we consider any movement to be good. If movement can be made, change can take place. Every individual has their own starting point. They have their own physical history, their own structure, their own capabilities, and their own current limitations. However, all movement is good.

In OS, everyone starts at "good". From there, we begin Pressing RESET and we move to "better," and eventually to "best." Best would be optimal movement for that person given their body and the history it contains.

The Three Guiding Principles

There are three guidelines to Pressing RESET:

1. Breathe using the diaphragm.
2. Activate the vestibular system (a sensory system that creates the sense of balance and spatial orientation for the purpose of coordinating movement with balance).
3. Engage in contra-lateral, cross-lateral, or midline crossing movements.

These three pillars are preprogrammed into each of our nervous systems and woven into the developmental sequence, the movements we flowed through as children.

It might seem strange, but the developmental sequence can actually develop in us at any age and any stage of our lives. The five developmental movements we are going to remember how to do are:

1. Belly Breathing
2. Learning to control the movement of our eyes and head
3. Rolling
4. Rocking
5. Crawling

These simple movements are the key to restoring our Original Strength, and in the subsequent pages, you will come to understand why we believe Original Strength and its Movement System - Pressing RESET - is an ideal approach for people with Parkinson's. It can serve as a stand-alone movement system or be a perfect complement to any other movement routines or programs you may practice.

Yes, movement is medicine, and the sooner the intervention the better! So, let's get started and learn how to Press RESET!

Pressing
RESET

RESET #1

Belly Breathing

THE VERY BEGINNING OF STRENGTH

Why?

- Learning to breathe deeply and fully can help with shallow breathing common to those with PD. It can also help a person with dyskinesia which sometimes causes rapid jerks in breathing rhythm.

- Due to a lack of dopamine, people with Parkinson's often struggle with anxiety and depression. Belly breathing calms your nervous system, soothes your emotions and allows you to think more clearly, helping you to manage stress and anxiety.

- You were born a "belly breather" and breathing through your diaphragm (your main breathing muscle) can promote improved posture that has been impaired by PD.

- It also helps to protect your spine and promote better movement.

How?

- This can be done from a variety of positions, but in the interest of brevity, we will explore two of these.

- If you are unable to get on the floor, you can do this sitting in the chair as illustrated in Position #2.

Position #1

BELLY BREATHING - LAYING ON YOUR BACK ON THE FLOOR HUGGING KNEES INTO THE CHEST. THIS CAN ALSO BE DONE ON YOUR MATTRESS IF YOU HAVE DIFFICULTY GETTING ON THE FLOOR.

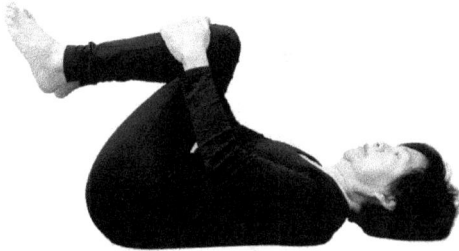

- Lie in this position.
- Place your tongue on the roof of your mouth and close your lips.
- Breathe in and out of your nose pulling air deep into your belly.

Position #2

BELLY BREATHING IN A CHAIR

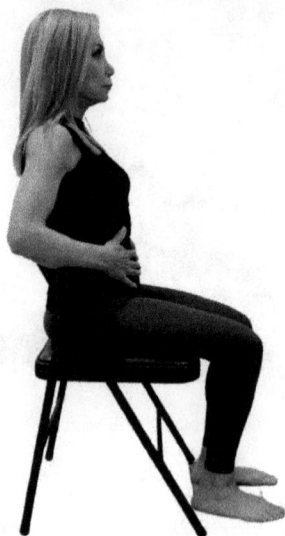

- Sit up tall with shoulders back and down and place your hands on your belly for tactile feedback.
- Place your tongue on the roof of your mouth and close your lips.
- Breathe in and out of your nose and pull air deep into your belly.

Head Control – The next layer of strength

Why?

- Parkinson's presents with balance, coordination, and postural challenges, as well as proprioception issues. These simple head control movements activate your vestibular system. This is your balance system and your sensory information collection point.

- Controlling the movements of your head can promote better balance, improve coordination and help to improve the constricted range of motion that you may be experiencing.

- People with Parkinson's can often feel that they've lost control of their bodies, but every muscle in your body is connected to the movements of your head. Therefore, the better you can control your head, the better you can control your entire body.

How?

There are many different positions that can be utilized.

Position #1

**CHIN TUCK – LAYING ON THE FLOOR OR ON YOUR MAT-
TRESS IF YOU HAVE DIFFICULTY GETTING ON THE FLOOR.**

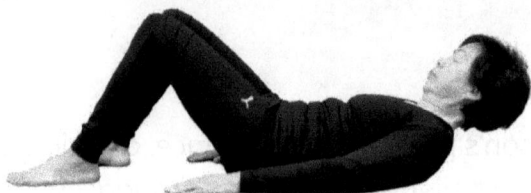

- Lie on your back on the floor (or on your mattress) in this position with knees bent and feet on the floor.

- Place your tongue on the roof of your mouth and close your lips.

- Raise your head by tucking your chin to your throat and lifting your head off the ground as if to look through your knees then slowly lower and repeat.

- Lead the movement with your eyes and look through your knees as you keep breathing through your nose.

CHIN TUCK – CHAIR VERSION

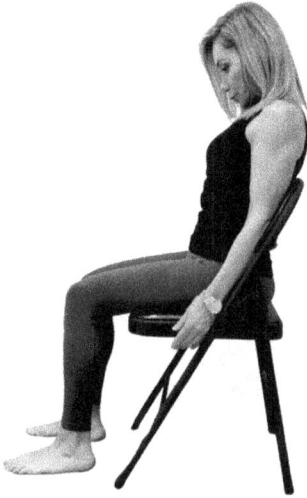

- Sit up tall in your chair.

- Place your tongue on the roof of your mouth and close your lips.

- Raise your head by tucking your chin to your throat while looking down. Then slowly bring your head back to neutral position and repeat.

- Lead the movement with your eyes.

- Do not hold your breath. Keep breathing through your nose.

Position #2

HEAD NOD

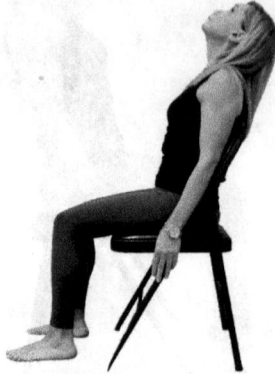

- Sit up tall in your chair or come onto the floor on all fours.
- Place your tongue on the roof of your mouth and close your lips.
- Perform head nods by raising and lowering your head as far back as your neck will allow you to move without moving into pain.
- Lead the movement with your eyes, looking toward the ceiling and then back to neutral position and repeat.
- Do not hold your breath. Keep breathing through your nose.

Pressing RESET for the Parkinson's Warrior

Rolling

Why?

- Balance challenges, slowness of movement and limb stiffness are prominent PD motor skill symptoms. Rolling can promote more fluidity of movement and help to reduce joint stiffness.

- Rolling can further improve and strengthen balance, one of the most difficult challenges for those with PD.

- Rolling also nourishes your spine and allows you to move more fluidly and effortlessly.

How?

Position #1

THE EGG ROLL

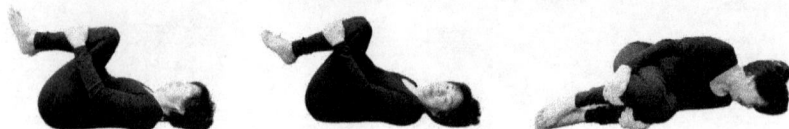

- Lie on your back either on the floor or on your mattress and grab your shins, hugging your knees into your chest.

- Maintain your belly breathing, mouth closed and tongue on the roof of your mouth.

- Lead with your eyes, look right, rotate your head to the right, then rotate your body to the right. Continue to look as far to the right as your body will allow.

- Keep holding onto your shins and just let your knees naturally gravitate to the floor.

- Then look left, rotate your head to the left, then rotate your body to the left. Continue to look as far to the left as your body will allow.

Pressing RESET for the Parkinson's Warrior

Rocking

Why?

- Rocking is another great movement for dealing with anxiety associated with Parkinson's. It soothes the nervous system.

- Rocking also helps to promote a healthy walking gait and improved posture which can be impaired by PD.

- It articulates the joints in a safe and easy way to help alleviate stiffness associated with PD.

- Rocking further nourishes the brain and coordinates the shoulders and hips preparing them for walking.

How?

Position #1

ON YOUR HANDS AND KNEES

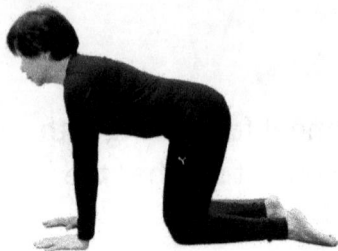

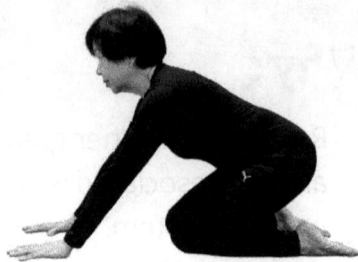

- Lips closed, nasal breathing, tongue on the roof of your mouth.
- Hold your head up and keep your eyes on the horizon.
- Keep your arms straight under your shoulders.
- Rock as far back as you can get to your heels.
- Now rock forward holding your chest proud until your chest is lined up with your hands.
- Keep your head and eyes on the horizon.

Position #2

THE ROCKING CHAIR

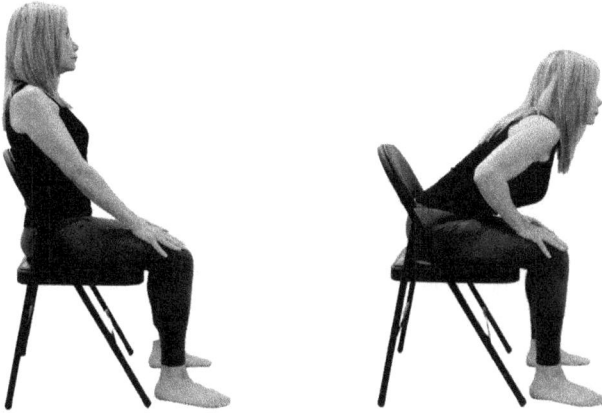

- Sit up nice and tall with lips closed, nasal breathing, head up on the horizon.

- Place your hands palms down on your thighs right above your knees.

- Simply rock forward as far as you can go while maintaining a proud chest and keeping your eyes on the horizon.

- Then rock all the way back until your back and shoulders are flush against the back of the chair and your shoulders are back and down.

- As always, keep your core braced throughout this reset.

RESET #5

RESET #5

Crawling – also known as contra-lateral movement

Why?

- Parkinson's is categorized as a "movement disorder" which is often expressed in an unhealthy walking gait as well as postural issues, slowness and joint stiffness.

- Crawling resets can be done even if you can't get on the floor. They can start in a chair or be done standing.

- Crawling connects both halves of the brain together, making it healthier and more efficient and reflexively connects the entire body and ties it together.

- If your walking gait has been impacted by PD, crawling can help to promote a healthier walking gait by making it more efficient and graceful.

How?

- Once again there are many variations, but we will start with Cross-Crawls and explore floor crawling as we move forward.

Position #1

STANDING CROSS CRAWLS

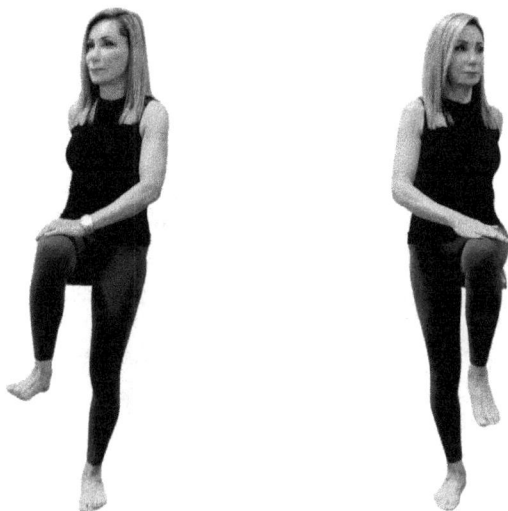

- Stand up nice and tall, shoulders back and down, core braced, lips closed, nasal breathing, tongue on the roof of the mouth.

- Touch your right hand to your left knee and touch your left hand to your right knee.

- This movement will help to open up your hips and help to foster a healthy walking gait.

- As it gets easier you can get more and more range of motion by tapping your opposite forearms to knees and eventually take your opposite elbows to opposite knees.

Position #2

CHAIR CROSS CRAWLS

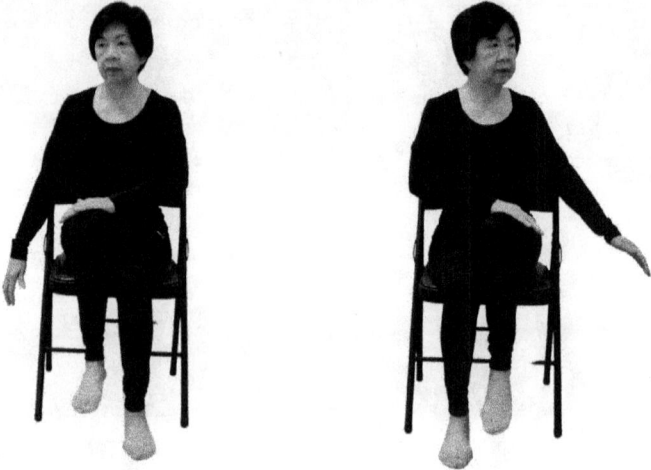

- Simply follow all of the instructions in the standing version but execute the movements while you are seated.

Position #3

CRAWLING ON THE FLOOR

Why?

- As stated above, crawling connects both halves of the brain together, making it healthier and more efficient.
- Crawling reflexively connects the body and ties it together.
- It strengthens the nervous system.

How?

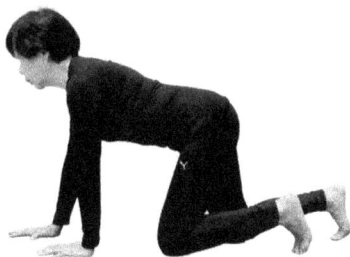

- Get on your hands and knees.
- Put your tongue on the roof of your mouth and practice your nasal breathing.
- Hold your head up and keep your eyes on the horizon. Keep a tall sternum and a proud chest.
- Move your opposite arms and legs together and crawl forward and backward.

PD Friendly Get Ups

Position #1

THE SIT TO STAND WITH ARM MOVEMENTS

Why?

- Getting up out of a chair and on and off the floor are critical movement patterns for anyone with PD that wants to maintain independence.

- These movements can help to strengthen legs, glutes and core when done with good form.

- Because Parkinson's tends to shrink and constrict movement, we have incorporated upper body "big" arm movements.

How?

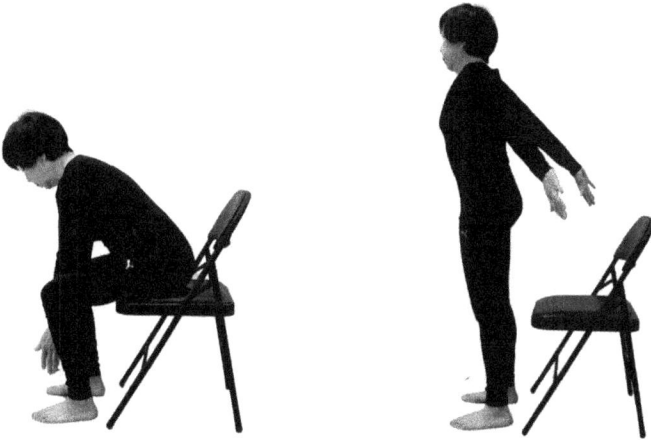

- Sit up tall with your feet hip width apart.

- Scoot forward slightly in your chair.

- Your heels should be lined up slightly behind your knees.

- Brace the core as you lean forward in the chair with fingertips towards the floor.

- Dig your heels into the floor as you rise up from the chair.

- Swing your arms up and out to the side pressing palms back with a slight pinch between the shoulder blades engaging upper back muscles.

- Sit back down and repeat.

Position #2

GETTING UP AND DOWN FROM THE FLOOR USING A CHAIR

Why?

- Similarly, this position will help you get onto the floor and up from the floor without assistance and it will ultimately make you feel safer and more secure once you master it.

- If done in multiple repetitions and at a good pace it will also elevate your heart rate and help to build endurance.

- It will help you to maintain mobility and independence.

How?

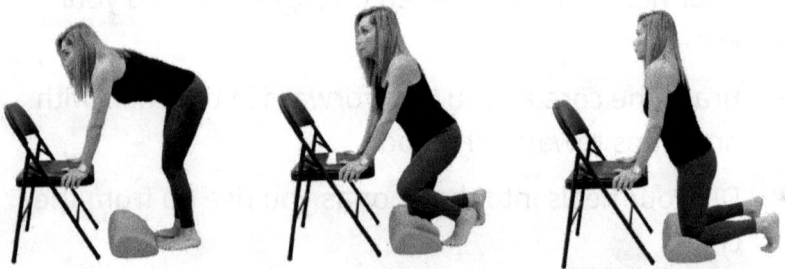

- Position yourself in front of a sturdy chair and place a small pillow in front of the chair to protect your knees if you are on a hard surface.

- Place your hands on the chair as you hinge at the waist with your feet aligned right behind the pillow.
- Bend one knee and place it on the pillow or floor.
- Bend the other knee and place it on the pillow or floor.
- Now do the opposite, put one heel back on the floor, and then the other heel on the floor, as you press your palms into the chair and stand up.
- This will bring you to your starting position.
- Now start all over and keep going down/down and up/up.

RESET #7

Smiling

Why?

- Dopamine loss is part of Parkinson's reality. Just like exercise, smiling can help to release higher levels of dopamine.

- Smiling places your nervous system at ease and sends the message, "I am safe," to the rest of your body.

- Smiling can boost the immune system and lower stress and blood pressure.

- Smiling feels good to the soul and the body.

- For people with Parkinson's who can lose expression in the facial muscles, smiling will recruit those facial muscles and encourage expression.

How?

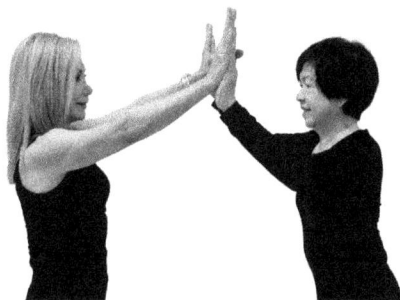

- Just smile from your lips, your eyes and your heart!
- Maintain the same number of repetitions as you are doing with the other resets.
- **Spend as much time as possible with people and things that make you smile.**

There is a very wide range of possible stages of PD but just know the more you deliberately move your body the better. Some of you may be athletic; some of you may be chair bound. Others will represent everything in between. You may need to gauge with support from a friend, care-partner or professional, which resets are best suited for you.

Additionally, we want to reinforce that even if you are already involved in other movement activities including Parkinson's Specific Programs, these resets will complement and enhance other movement activities effectively.

Your
DESIGN

The Power in Your Design

Based on the way a diagnosis of Parkinson's is typically communicated, it is understandable that people with Parkinson's can feel powerless and even at war with their bodies.

After all, it is explained as a definitive prognosis and can evoke feelings of fear and anxiety. Thankfully today, the best Parkinson's Movement Disorder Specialists are now prescribing early and consistent movement intervention. This makes all the difference in how well people living with PD will fare. Just knowing that you can do something about your circumstances to control the outcome can alleviate some of the negative emotions and propel you to take action.

We want you to take that a step further; our intention is to provide you with a new and hopeful perspective and to give you an opportunity to take control through movement restoration and explain how it occurs. Knowing the "why" and "how" can bolster your belief system, creating a more positive and desirable approach. We want you to know that the hope of healing and the expression of strength already live inside your nervous system and give you the means to successfully tap into it. Your very design contains the movement program intended to keep you strong, able and healthy.

Spending just a few minutes every day relearning or remembering how to do these movements will enable you to live better and more independently. It will help you to reclaim strength and health and to live your best life.

Staying positive, being patient with yourself and loving yourself enough to invest in the time with consistent effort will help you to rediscover your Original Strength. **It's your move...**

Simple Daily Restoration Plan

Perform the routine 1-3 times as follows:

1. Belly breathing – 2-3 minutes

    Either laying on the floor, holding knees into chest or knees bent with feet on the floor; or seated or standing. Choose your position, breathing in and out through your nose, keeping your tongue on the roof of your mouth. Focus on pulling air deep down into your belly. It may help to imagine trying to pull air down to your feet.

    Why?

    Because this is where change starts. Breathing with your diaphragm makes you solid in your center and it helps your body work at optimum hormone levels. It keeps you in "peace and harmony" mode and out of "fight, flight and panic mode."

2. Head nods – 1 minute

    Choose whatever position you feel most comfortable in - seated, standing or on all fours in a tabletop position. Lift your head up looking at the ceiling as far as your head will let you move without moving into pain. Then move back to a neutral position.

Why?

Because every muscle in your body is connected to the movements of your head. The body is designed to follow the head. Remembering how to move your head will, in a sense, sharpen and improve all the reflexive connections from your head to the rest of your body. This can help restore your reflexive strength.

3. Rolling around on the floor – 3 minutes

If getting up and down on the floor is easily accessible to you, roll any way you want to roll for three minutes. You can start with egg rolls as illustrated in the booklet. Lead with your eyes and head when rolling. If you get dizzy, try slowing down or reducing the range of motion of your rolls.

Why?

Rolling sharpens your balance and feeds your brain with rich nourishment; it makes your brain healthier. Rolling also connects your center, layering more strength on top of the solid foundation the diaphragmatic breathing started. Rolling prepares your body to coordinate more complex movements.

4. Rocking on Hands and Knees – 3 minutes

Keep your head up, stay "proud" in your chest and rock your butt back towards your feet for three minutes. Rock back as far as you can go while maintaining a strong chest. DO NOT move into pain. If the floor is not accessible to you, practice the chair version illustrated in the booklet.

Why?

Because rocking integrates all of the major moving joints of your body. It makes you whole and prepares your body to move gracefully while soothing your nervous system and your emotions. Rocking also sets and restores posture.

5. Cross-Crawling – 3 minutes

Touch your opposite limbs together alternating for three minutes. They should move fluidly, together. That is, your right arm should move along with and at the same time as your left leg. Breathe in and out through your nose and keep your mouth closed.

Why?

Because cross-crawling is the simplest engagement of your gait pattern (walking). It's also the movement that can tie your brain together and connect your whole body. It can make you whole in both brain and body.

6. Get Ups (getting up and down from the floor) – 2-3 minutes

Practice moving from the ground to standing. If you have no balance challenges, lie down on the floor and stand up. Repeat and do this in as many ways as you can think of - be creative. If you need assistance, use the PD Friendly Get Up shown in this booklet and don't forget to practice your "sit to stands" getting in and out of the chair.

Why?

Your ability to get up and down easily will improve your longevity and your quality of life while maintaining your independence. We must always master our bodies' movements and resist gravity with ease to maintain our resiliency.

That's it. It's about 15 minutes of gentle movement and covers all the fundamentals to help you improve your strength, balance and mobility.

The 3 Minute Calming Reset

This routine is appropriate for everyone and by now you know how important it is for people with PD to practice movement daily or as frequently as possible, but we know that life can sometimes get in the way. This simple 3-minute routine is also a great way to start your day, especially if you have difficulty getting on the floor without help. You can do the first two movements on your mattress and then get up and do the cross crawls standing or even sitting on the edge of your bed. This will help to alleviate the stiffness that often occurs upon rising.

This is also an ideal movement sequence to use if you are having a hectic day or you are feeling anxious or stressed at any time - find three minutes, and complete the following routine.

1. **Breathe with your diaphragm (belly breathing) x 1 minute**

   You can do this anywhere at any time and it will calm you down and take you out of "fight or flight mode". As mentioned earlier in the book this will also address the shallow breathing that is a common symptom of Parkinson's.

   Close your lips and place your tongue in its natural position on the roof of your mouth. Take big deep breaths into your belly, inhaling and exhaling through the nose. You can place your hands on your belly to feel it expand so that you know you are doing it correctly.

2. **Rock back and forth x 1 minute**

   Get on your hands and knees in a table-top position. Keep your chest proud and your head looking up on the horizon. Maintain your belly breathing and tongue on the roof of your mouth. We have seen clients increase their range of motion considerably with regular practice of this movement.

   Remember to maintain your gaze up on the horizon as you rock back to your heels and then back to the original table-top position.

   Chair Modification:

   Simply place your hands on your knees and rock your chest towards your lap and then back into place sitting up tall. Keep your gaze and head up on the horizon for the entire exercise.

3. **Standing or seated cross-crawls x 1 minute**

   Touch your opposite limbs together, moving back and forth from side to side. Touch wherever you can comfortably reach - hand to knee, forearm to knee, or elbow to knee for the most advanced method. If done regularly, this exercise will help alleviate some of the stiffness in hips and lower back often associated with Parkinson's.

This simple 3-minute routine will leave you feeling calmer, energized and less stiff. You will be glad you took the time!

Featured in the Pictures

Lorna Castaneda

In the pictures throughout this booklet are the author, Ginny, with Lorna. Lorna is a 76-year-old Parkinson's Warrior! Upon her diagnosis at age 70, Lorna vowed that she would do what she needed to do to maintain her health and not allow PD to hinder her zest for life.

"I am going to do everything possible to slow down the progression."

In doing so Lorna takes a very consistent and holistic approach to her health and well-being, ensuring that she is engaging her mind and body, and feeding her spirit with activities that bring her joy.

Lorna's interests are plentiful. She is a world-traveler, participates in a variety of movement programs and activities, plays the piano and takes singing lessons to keep her voice strong. We hope she will inspire others to remain active and to pursue their individual goals and passions.

Want to learn more?

This booklet was designed to give a brief overview of the Original Strength System and how it can help you Press RESET to become a stronger Warrior in your fight with Parkinson's.

We put it together because we know it can help everyone and anyone. If you do nothing more than what is in this booklet, you will notice many changes in how your mind and body begin to feel and react to various situations.

Original Strength is a human movement education company with a mission to bring the hope and strength of movement to every body in the world. Based on the human developmental sequence and the human body's design, the Original Strength System teaches movements that help RESET an individual's neuromuscular system, allowing them to enjoy improved physical movement and physiological function.

We conduct courses, training, and certify coaches and instructors. We also develop educational materials for PE teachers, physical therapy students, medical professionals, trainers, coaches fitness/health/wellness instructors, sports conditioning professionals, and individuals/groups working with vestibular and neuromuscular functionality.

If you want to know more about Pressing RESET and regaining your original strength, visit https://

originalstrength.net. There you will find a variety of books, hundreds of free video tutorials (**OS Movement Snax**), and a complete listing of our courses and OS Certified Professionals near you.

You may want to consider finding an OS Certified Professional. These professionals will conduct an Original Strength Screen and Assessment (OSSA), which is the quickest and easiest way to identify areas your movement system needs to go from good to best. The OSSA allows a pro to pinpoint the best place for you to start Pressing RESET and restoring your Original Strength.

We encourage you to reach out to the OS team with any questions you may have. ***Please keep us updated with your progress; we really want to know how you are doing - progress@OriginalStrength.net.***

Press RESET now and live life better & stronger because you were awesomely and wonderfully made to accomplish amazing things.

For more information:

⏻riginal
strength

Original Strength Systems, LLC
OriginalStrength.net

PressingRESETfor@Originalstrength.net

original
strength

originalstrength.net

Published by

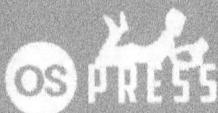 OS PRESS